Into remission from overwhelming fatigue

This book is difficult to categorise, as it is based on both personal experiences and the latest medical research. It can also be considered to be a self-help book in some ways.

In the past, Frank had a definite "web presence" and operated a small number of websites. However, that activity has been abandoned as it proved to be very time consuming, and counterproductive to some extent. At the moment, he only has limited involvement in a chronic fatigue syndrome (CFS) web forum, and a melanoma research website.

Since being diagnosed with CFS, it has been Frank's heartfelt wish to help other sufferers to overcome this poorly understood physical illness. It is hoped that anyone battling CFS will find this book of some value.

Frank's son Nick has also included his insights on the profoundly insidious effects that CFS has had on family life since he was a young child.

INTO REMISSION FROM OVERWHELMING FATIGUE

Frank Bartosy, Nick Bartosy

First published by Busybird Publishing 2020

Copyright © 2020 Frank Bartosy and Nick Bartosy

ISBN

PRINT 978-1-922465-00-9

EBOOK 978-1-922465-01-6

This work is copyright. Apart from any use permitted under the Copyright Act 1968, no part of this publication may be reproduced, stored in a retrieval system or transmitted in any form or by any means, electronic, mechanical, photocopying, recording or otherwise, without the prior written permission of Frank Bartosy and Nick Bartosy.

Cover Image: Nick Bartosy

Layout and typesetting: Busybird Publishing

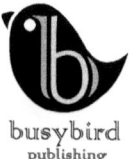

Busybird Publishing
2/118 Para Road
Montmorency, Victoria
Australia 3094

Disclaimer: The information in this book is based on personal experiences, new research and unproven treatments. There can be no guarantees that other people will benefit from the information provided. Any research and opinions within the text are taken from personal experience and the resources listed at the back of the book.

The authors are not medical practitioners and cannot accept any form of liability or responsibility, legal or otherwise, if the material in this book adversely influences any person's individual state of health.

It is suggested that a competent and qualified medical doctor should closely supervise all medical treatments.

This book aims to dispel the widespread prejudicial belief that CFS is a permanent illness that cannot possibly be overcome.

Contents

About the authors	1
Acknowledgements	3
Foreword	5
Chapter 1 The strangest disease	7
Chapter 2 Chronic fatigue syndrome and fibromyalgia	17
Chapter 3 Diagnosis, mechanisms, probiotics and stages of CFS	21
Chapter 4 The situation changes	39
Chapter 5 My experience living with a CFS sufferer	47
Conclusion	51
References	53
Index	57

About the authors

Frank's interest in the areas of health, fitness and nutrition developed over the long time that he spent studying the martial arts. In particular he was intrigued by the role that optimum nutrition could play in helping people achieve robust health and a high level of physical fitness.

After achieving the rank of second Dan black belt in taekwondo, he qualified as a level 1 coach. Frank later became a government licensed taekwondo instructor. He then conducted classes in the suburbs of Chelsea and The Patch in Melbourne, Australia.

In 1993, while employed as a Principal Technical Officer with Telstra, Frank's health started to deteriorate. He was eventually diagnosed with post viral syndrome (PVS) in 1994.

By early 1997, Frank had made virtually no progress in trying to regain his health. However, in late 1997 Frank discovered that he was severely deficient in essential fatty acids. Supplementation with fish, flax and evening primrose oils gave him a significant level of improvement in his condition.

Despite experiencing a noticeable level of amelioration in most symptoms, he was unable to return to full-time work. This placed an enormous strain on his family's finances, as Frank was the only breadwinner. In addition to paying off a mortgage he was supporting his wife, Rosy and their young son, Nick.

Frank appreciates Nick's offer to contribute to this book. Like Frank, he has been challenged by having to endure the trauma of Rosy's cancer treatment and tragic death.

Despite this situation, Nick has courageously managed to graduate from university with a Bachelor of Business and Commerce, majoring in marketing.

He has consequently worked at a major sports stadium for a long time and hopes to continue serving his customers throughout the forthcoming football and cricket seasons.

Acknowledgements

We would like to thank many people who helped make this book possible. They are listed below in approximate alphabetical order:

Dr Zev Barr. His continued encouragement since Frank's diagnosis is greatly appreciated.

Judy Bartosy. Frank's mum and published writer. She introduced him to Busybird Publishing as he provided her with IT support. This resulted in Judy's manuscript of *My Journey to Freedom* being published.

Nancy Brown. Frank's mother in-law whose support has made this book possible.

Rob Hepworth. A skilful proofreader and great friend.

The people from the original Bioscreen research team.

Dr Jacob Teitelbaum. Without his article about treating CFS with statins, we wouldn't have attempted this book.

Foreword

Since the book *Your victory over chronic fatigue syndrome* was published, Frank undeniably experienced a short remission of some symptoms. Unfortunately, his beloved wife Rosy was diagnosed with metastatic melanoma in 2007 and the resultant stress gradually triggered a relapse of CFS.

The situation undoubtedly left Frank and his family in an environment of chronic and unrelenting stress. It is known that CFS sufferers have a great deal of difficulty dealing with stress because of the way hormones are affected by the disease. So, it is not surprising that CFS returned while Rosy fought the devastating effects of cancer and treatment side effects.

Frank remained moderately affected until 2012, when he experienced another mild remission that wasn't truly comprehensive in nature. He relapsed again some months later, and was experiencing a slow deterioration in his health until things changed dramatically in September 2019.

1

The strangest disease

Chronic fatigue syndrome (CFS) is, quite possibly, the strangest disease imaginable. The fact that experts still can't agree on one universally accepted term for this condition highlights the mysterious nature of CFS.[1] It is also commonly referred to as post viral syndrome (PVS), myalgic encephalomyelitis (ME), chronic fatigue immune dysfunction syndrome (CFIDS) or systemic exertion intolerance disease (SEID).

While it is appreciated that fibromyalgia syndrome (FMS) is often viewed as an unrelated condition, the authors believe that this is incorrect. They feel that FMS is a special type of CFS in which chronic pain is the major symptom.

Chronic fatigue syndrome (CFS) is a term that has become the most widely accepted general name for long-term fatigue related disorders in Australia. Although this is an inaccurate way to describe the serious nature of this illness, it appears that we are stuck with it!

Therefore, the remainder of this book will often use the term chronic fatigue syndrome as a general term for the conditions mentioned above. Where necessary, the expression chronic fatigue/pain disorder may also be used.

What are chronic fatigue/pain disorders?

Chronic fatigue/pain disorders are a range of illnesses that have long-term fatigue and/or pain as their major symptoms. Often there is no history of the sufferer experiencing a physical injury, and pain appears to be related to a chronic infection. Until recently, medical science has been confounded by the range of seemingly inexplicable symptoms that are present in many cases of these illnesses.

Australia's pioneering Bioscreen research team gave a presentation at the 1998 Sydney CFS Conference called *Host versus acquired responses in defined CFS patients*. The researchers put forward their belief that the use of CFS as a clinical diagnosis is not supported by the available data and should be replaced with the diagnosis of a chronic fatigue disorder [2].

As a result of these research findings, the term has been expanded to include myalgia or pain symptoms. The expression chronic fatigue/pain disorder has virtually replaced all previous names for these illnesses in Bioscreen literature.

In more recent years, the original research personnel from the Bioscreen team have been involved in variety of other projects.

Symptoms of chronic fatigue/pain disorders

Chronic fatigue/pain disorders are serious long-term illnesses that can last a lifetime. These conditions have symptoms that can often be similar to other illnesses. Left untreated, some patients may improve somewhat over time. Others may get better, and then experience a relapse. This pattern is sometimes repeated a number of times in a cyclical manner.

A small proportion of people may experience progressive deterioration. Although it is very rare for any fatal cases to be officially recognised, the serious effects that an illness such as this can have on one's life should never be taken lightly. It can lead to heart problems and other conditions that can significantly reduce life expectancy.

Many sufferers will remain chronically ill and make little progress towards anything that could be considered as good health. At the present time, full recovery from these illnesses tends to be a very rare occurrence.

CFS/FMS has been found to have a number of similar characteristics to cases of influenza or glandular fever.

These similarities can include:

- Mild fever.
- Swollen lymph nodes (also known as glands).
- Profound lethargy or tiredness.
- Generalised body aches and pains.
- Sore throat.

Despite these similarities, there are also significant differences. It is now known that the Epstein-Barr virus is the cause of glandular fever, and can cause many symptoms that are similar to CFS. However, the cause of CFS has not been isolated to any particular viral or microbial infection.

Chronic fatigue disorders cause variable degrees of muscle fatigue and pain. The major symptoms that usually distinguish these illnesses from other diseases are:

- Intense levels of constant or recurring physical fatigue.
- A high susceptibility to mental exhaustion.
- Inability to concentrate or to think clearly for long periods.
- Muscle and/or joint pain.
- Generalised unexplained aches.
- Vague symptoms of chronic ill health.

Sensations of fatigue are often experienced at the slightest exertion, and can sometimes make people so debilitated that they are unable to get out of bed for extended periods of time. Indeed, some patients have described their illness as having symptoms of temporary muscular paralysis. This type of fatigue is very unlike that found in most other diseases. In fact, it is felt that physical and mental exhaustion is a much better way to describe this feeling. Some have more accurately defined this feeling as being like 'crushing fatigue' that is very different from ordinary tiredness.

If these symptoms persist for more than six months, the sufferer will normally be diagnosed by a doctor as suffering from PVS, ME, CFS, CFIDS, SEID and/or FMS. It is important to note that the illness is currently diagnosed on the basis of symptoms alone without the benefit of any specific pathology tests. Although there are various experimental tests available, these do not as yet meet the standards of the orthodox medical establishment.

Other clinical features of CFS may include gastrointestinal symptoms, short-term memory problems, headaches, very dry skin and slow wound healing. In chronic fatigue syndrome, the immune system certainly appears to be malfunctioning. There is some evidence that it is "chronically overactive" and dysregulated in subtle ways. Sufferers often find that it takes much longer than healthy people do to overcome infections. It is common for CFS patients to take more than three weeks to overcome a bout of the common cold. Other people usually overcome this illness in about one week.

Undeniably, chronic fatigue syndrome does have many of the characteristics that other chronic illnesses share. These include long term adverse effects that may eventually harm the sufferer's physical and psychological well-being. Some examples of these detrimental effects are loss of physical fitness, deconditioned muscles, weight problems, rejection by friends, relatives and even some doctors.

Early evidence

Despite appearing to be a modern disease, CFS has probably been around for well over 200 years. The earliest record of an illness that resembles CFS has been traced back to around 1750. The medical literature of the time described a condition named febricula, which had similar neurological and muscular symptoms to its present-day equivalent[3].

There have been claims made that prominent people such as Charles Darwin and Florence Nightingale may have had a type of chronic fatigue disorder. While there hasn't been much discovered about the nature of Charles Darwin's affliction, there is a strong chance that Florence Nightingale did have CFS.

There is evidence that she was stricken by a debilitating chronic illness. It appeared to have closely resembled a typical case of CFS. Despite having ill health that caused her to be virtually bedridden, she achieved a great deal and was responsible for establishing the first School of Nursing [3].

It was recently decided that May 12 should be chosen as International CFS Awareness Day in order to commemorate Florence Nightingale's birthday.

Recent outbreaks

Historically, medical literature didn't seem to pay much attention to CFS-like illnesses, probably due to the varied nature and apparent obscurity of the symptoms. It was not until 1934 that the illness achieved prominence in the United States.

CFS in the United States

In 1934, a debilitating disease badly affected the operation of the Los Angeles County General Hospital.

The outbreak involved the medical staff of the hospital, and caused initial worries that it was a polio outbreak.

Although the patients' muscles remained weak, there was no evidence of muscle wasting and therefore polio was ruled out as a cause. When the victims of this mysterious disease were thoroughly examined six months later, over half continued to remain unwell.

Further small outbreaks continued to occur, but there was no prominent occurrence until fairly recent times. In 1985, a mysterious disease that caused many people to have chronic flu-like symptoms struck the town of Lake Tahoe Nevada. Extensive media interest was raised, and the disease soon came to be known as the yuppie flu. Despite having little evidence on the actual cause of this outbreak, the term chronic Epstein-Barr virus was invented to satisfy demands that the illness be given a legitimate name.

Subsequently, a national organisation was formed with many people believing that a type of Epstein-Barr virus had caused this illness. Eventually, some patients recovered but most remained chronically affected by the illness to some extent.

CFS in Great Britain: "The Royal Free" disease

In 1955, the Royal Free Hospital in London admitted large numbers of people who had been affected by a disease that had experts bewildered. It appeared to be the start of a serious, large-scale epidemic in this area of London.

The major symptoms consisted of muscular fatigue and neurological disturbances that followed an initial acute infection. Although resembling polio in many ways, the inconsistent symptoms did not match any known disease.

With numerous medical staff as well the patients being

affected, the hospital could no longer cope with the workload. Consequently, it was decided that the hospital had little option but to close for some months.

When the epidemic subsided and the Royal Free hospital was again operational, only a small number of victims had recovered. Unfortunately, a large proportion of people affected by this outbreak became chronically ill.

Much interest was initially raised in the cause of this baffling illness, that later became known as the Royal Free disease. Further research suggested that the name myalgic encephalomyelitis (ME) would be a more accurate description of this mysterious sickness.

When extensive medical tests failed to find the cause of the outbreak, many doctors eventually became sceptical about the organic nature of the disease. Indeed, claims have since been made by psychiatrists in the UK that the illness was due to an episode of mass hysteria!

This has resulted in many doctors forming the opinion that such an illness was not real and therefore should not be taken seriously.

Other outbreaks of CFS

There have been numerous isolated outbreaks of CFS throughout the world. The epidemics in the UK and US demonstrate that significant and seemingly acute outbreaks of CFS may sometimes occur.

It now appears that most cases are geographically isolated from each other. While these seem to be random occurrences, it is difficult to be certain of anything to do with CFS. So it isn't surprising that there has been very little in the way of statistical information that has been accurately collected and analysed.

Indeed, the authors now believe that factors such as one's genetics and diet may play a significant role in the disease process. It is possible that the types of food and drink consumed could affect the likely prognosis of each individual.

Intriguingly, there have been very few reports of CFS-like medical conditions in developing countries. While doctors in these regions are normally concerned in dealing with more acute and conspicuous illnesses, it is felt that this fact is noteworthy. It gives us a clue that helps to pinpoint one factor that could be important in the explaining why some people succumb to CFS.

2

Chronic fatigue syndrome and fibromyalgia

Symptoms and signs

A special type of crushing fatigue, unlike that found in most other diseases is often a central feature of chronic fatigue/pain disorders. With the typical CFS patient, an almost immediate sensation of muscular fatigue and some pain will follow any physical activity that is perceived as being too strenuous.

This type of fatigue referred to by sufferers of CFS is difficult to describe, but is similar to the feeling of experiencing total physical and mental exhaustion. On reaching this point, the patient has no choice but to stop all activity and rest. In severe cases, the sufferer will be forced to take some hours of immediate bedrest before they can recover sufficient energy to resume daily life.

Disturbingly, this critical threshold point of exhaustion can occur whilst undertaking the most trivial amount of physical activity such as walking around the block, or simply just doing very light housework!

Obviously, this can occur at times that in the early stages of severe CFS can be very unpredictable. However, if one is aware of how energy levels can fluctuate throughout the day a clearer picture of when this is likely to happen can be obtained.

It is accepted that normal people have energy levels that fluctuate over the course of a typical day. Many healthy individuals find that they have a decline in their energy levels after lunch. By mid-afternoon, this feeling will normally be overcome with energy restored to acceptable levels.

However, many CFS patients are forced to have a period of bedrest after midday. In more severe cases, sufferers experience a slump in energy levels that take hours to overcome. So, instead of experiencing a recovery by mid-afternoon many CFS sufferers may not recover until the evening. Indeed, there is now some evidence that the body's natural circadian rhythms can be severely disrupted by CFS.

It is important to note that the need for the patient to have a period of bedrest has nothing do with the desire to sleep. Frank remembers that people will think that if one has to lie down, it is assumed that this is because one is sleepy. However, Frank has always felt that the sensation of overwhelming muscle fatigue was the sole reason for him having daily bedrest.

It is interesting to note that sufferers afflicted by severe CFS may, at times, find even simple tasks such as standing or sitting upright difficult. As these actions involve the use of a degree of muscular effort, a patient who has run out of energy will feel exhausted. They may not be physically able to stand up without great difficulty. This problem is certainly not limited to the major muscle groups, and it is felt that other parts of the body can also be affected. It is this fact that gives us a hint as to how CFS affects the energy metabolism at a cellular level.

It may not be obvious that the muscles involved in vision can often be affected by chronic fatigue syndrome. This means that sufferers can find reading difficult, as their eye muscles can become easily fatigued. When fatigue sets in, text will appear indistinct as focusing will become an increasingly difficult task. Although this symptom may be distressing, if it is due to CFS it is only temporary. Obviously, if it is suspected that the vision problem may be due to another cause, medical and/or optical advice should be sought.

It is interesting that mental tasks that require periods of concentration such as reading, writing and performing mathematical calculations can also cause significant levels of physical fatigue. This feeling is often called brain fog and is similar to how people feel when they are suffering from influenza, and at the same time trying to carry out exacting intellectual work.

Another way to look at the fatigue experienced in CFS is to assume that sufferers have a limited amount of energy that they can expend without difficulty. In contrast, normal healthy individuals are not troubled by this concern until they overexert themselves for long periods.

When this level of overexertion takes place, healthy people will usually need a few minutes to recover. In contrast, CFS patients can take many hours to recover from activity. In severe cases, the victims of CFS may take days to regain their limited level of available energy. In fact, it is likely that severe exertion will cause a relapse in many CFS symptoms and increase the chances of a serious deterioration in the patient's condition.

When muscles have been overworked, the CFS patient may find it difficult to move them at all. It may feel like one's limbs are made out of lead, and that they have become too heavy to move! Yes, this is a very strange sensation indeed and healthy people will find it difficult to believe that one can actually feel this way.

Perhaps it is no wonder that doctors have thought that some CFS cases were caused by a polio-like virus that caused symptoms of temporary paralysis. Indeed, one can speculate that it was this idea that prompted researchers to assume that CFS must be caused by a specific virus.

3

Diagnosis, mechanisms, probiotics and stages of CFS

The Centers for Disease Control and Prevention (CDC) in Atlanta initially devised definitions of chronic fatigue syndrome for researchers. The basic diagnostic criteria for CFS in the USA were consequently based on these CDC guidelines. At the time when these criteria were first created, it was assumed that chronic fatigue syndrome was an infectious disease of unknown cause[9] [10].

Therefore, as there was no diagnostic test that could accurately identify CFS as a distinct illness, scientific and medical experts were left with a fairly imprecise set of parameters to follow. Since the CDC Atlanta criteria have been adopted by doctors as the basis on which most CFS cases are currently diagnosed, there remains considerable scope for confusion and misdiagnosis. The major problem is that the doctors are compelled to give a definite diagnosis on the basis of symptoms alone. It is also assumed that all other likely causes of fatigue have been considered and eliminated as the source of the symptoms[3].

In other words, many patients who have been evaluated in strict accordance to the CDC criteria may actually have a number of diseases or disorders that go under the general definition of chronic fatigue syndrome.

It is felt that CFS now should be considered to be a general term that covers illnesses in which chronic fatigue is the major symptom. It seems that it should no longer be simply considered as one infectious disease, as it was assumed when the CDC criteria were devised. Indeed, there is no significant evidence that chronic fatigue syndrome is definitely caused by any particular virus or microbial agent.

Instead, it is felt that CFS should be considered as a combination of known chronic disorders, genetic factors and dietary deficiencies.

It has recently been discovered that probiotics can influence symptom expression. There is ongoing research that has found that the gastrointestinal flora is altered in a specific way in CFS patients.

Some key terms[6]:

- Genome: The complete genetic information such as the DNA or RNA of an organism.

- Microbiome: The community of microbes within the human gut.
- Pathogenesis: The origin and development of a disease.
- Peripheral neuropathy: Disease of the nervous system affecting the ends of the nerve fibres.
- Virome: The genomes that are contained within an organism or environment.

What are the mechanisms involved in CFS?

This is a summary of Frank's current understanding of the biological processes involved in this baffling illness.

These mechanisms include:

- Impaired immune system due to gut barrier dysfunction[4].
- The consequences of exposure to toxins in some cases.
- Medical history and genetics.
- Altered lipid metabolism[4] associated with an abnormal requirement for essential fatty acids in some people.

- Myelin alterations possible due to abnormal lipid metabolism.[4]
- Abnormal glucose tolerance[4].
- Viral-induced microbiome changes[5].

It has recently been discovered that viruses are able to infect the bacterial microbiome. Viral-induced microbiome alterations consequently been found to have the ability to influence the CFS patient's health and prognosis.

As medical technology advances, it is becoming evident that the virome can affect host health, and may be involved in the pathogenesis of CFS. Further research in this field is clearly required if we are to understand the complex mechanisms involved in this enigmatic disease.

Frank's experience:

Frank's unusually high requirement for EFAs has resulted in him experiencing the likely effects of myelin changes. He has noticed that there is a problem with occasional mild peripheral neuropathy in both feet. It is felt that this confirms some of the recent research carried out by Dr Neil McGregor[4].

Dr McGregor has been involved in the study of CFS for a very long time and was involved in the work of the Bioscreen research team in the 1990s.

Probiotics

The pioneering Bioscreen research team highlighted the importance of gastrointestinal flora in the 1990s[2]. Their particular area of research was focused on chronic fatigue syndrome for a considerable length of time.

With this research in mind, Frank tried probiotics at various times during his illness. Unfortunately, they didn't help him very much at all. At times they even proved detrimental, as they increased the level of fatigue and brain fog that he was experiencing.

It was not until Frank read about the types of bacteria that were altered in chronic fatigue syndrome that the penny dropped – Frank was taking the wrong bacteria!

So, it appears that for the probiotic treatment concept to be useful it is very important to take the correct forms of bacteria. However, suitable formulations are not yet readily available (to the best of our knowledge at time of writing).

In addition, other types of bacteria should be somehow reduced. It is unclear how this can be achieved.

Researchers have recently discovered that differences in the levels of seven types of gut bacteria (Faecalibacterium, Roseburia, Dorea, Coprococcus, Clostridium, Coprobacillus and Ruminococcus) are strongly linked to CFS[7]. Clearly, more studies are required.

The stages of CFS

Although chronic fatigue syndrome usually appears to commence after the sufferer has had a triggering viral infection, it is felt that the CFS disease process often begins a long time before this infection occurs. In fact, it may begin months or years before symptoms become evident[1]. This process can be divided into four stages, as detailed in the following pages.

Stage 1

Mild EFA deficiencies cause vague symptoms of ill health

It has been recently discovered that essential fatty acid (EFA) deficiencies can cause immune system malfunctions. Recent scientific findings into essential fatty acids (EFAs) indicate that a healthy immune system must have sufficient levels of the right type of EFAs. It is thought that these play a major role in the chemical pathways that effect body's immune system and inflammation responses.

It is interesting to note that EFAs were once thought to be a type of vitamin. In fact, at least one book that we know about refers to vitamin F as an acceptable name for essential fatty acids. Perhaps EFAs should be considered to be as important as the common vitamins A, B, C and E that are so vital to our nutritional needs.

The latest research now states that the immune systems of people deficient in any type of EFA could have difficulties in fully overcoming many infections.

Alarmingly, evidence now points to the existence of widespread EFA deficiencies in parts of the general population[11]. Therefore, it is probable that nutritional deficiencies are largely responsible for contributing to the cause of a range chronic diseases and disorders, including CFS.

Symptoms of EFA deficiencies

There is, at the present time, a paucity of accurate information available on the symptoms of essential fatty acid deficiencies. However, the following conditions are thought to be good indicators of EFA deficiencies:

- extremely dry skin.
- susceptibility to infections.
- heart and circulation problems.
- behavioural problems.
- poor nail condition.
- intestinal problems.
- tiredness or fatigue.
- systemic inflammation.
- arthritis-like conditions.
- poor rate of wound healing.

Stage 2

EFA deficiencies and microbial infections cause an illness known as chronic fatigue (CF)

It has been found that the immune system releases chemicals such as cytokines and lymphokines in response to any infective agent. These chemicals are potentially toxic and are thought to be responsible for many of the symptoms of illnesses that accompany any infection.

The authors speculate that the primary infective agent need not be any specific virus and can be bacterial or fungal in nature. They now feel that any significant challenge to the immune system can trigger CFS in susceptible individuals. The challenges can include a variety of infections and exposure to toxic chemicals.

It is felt that the illness, colloquially referred to as chronic fatigue or CF is a precursor to chronic fatigue syndrome. It seems that the preliminary symptoms of chronic fatigue start to occur in this second stage of the CFS disease process. If left untreated, it is felt that CF will often lead to CFS.

It is often not recognised that bacterial infections can remain undetected, despite basic blood tests, and become a chronic health problem. The authors feel that germs such as staphylococci bacteria can play a significant part in the CFS disease process.

It is recognised that abscesses can occur in the gums, in bone, and in body organs such as the liver. If a hidden bacterial infection such as an abscess is present at a time when EFA levels are low, it is possible that continual amounts of microbial toxins, together with immune system chemicals will be released into the bloodstream. If the levels of cytokines, lymphokines and other toxins are permitted to build up in the bloodstream, a point will soon be reached where the affected person will start to feel ill, with vague symptoms.

The resultant symptoms will be similar to typical of cases of mild central nervous system chemical poisoning, and will be identical in nature to an indistinct illness where chronic fatigue is the main problem.

Therefore, it is proposed that chronic fatigue can be triggered by an infection or chemical toxin occurring at a time when omega 3 and other essential fatty acid levels are very low.

Frank's experience:

Before he was diagnosed with CFS, Frank had a period of some months during which he felt intermittent flu-like symptoms, together with feelings of abnormal tiredness. Frank noticed that his temperature was often in the region 37 -37.5 degrees C. The medical books that Frank read, said that this temperature range was all right, as the range from 36.5-37.5 degrees C was considered to be normal.

However, he knew that he was a little warm and it is now believed that he did have a mild fever in response to a chronic bacterial infection (dental abscess). Frank also had symptoms of EFA deficiencies such as dry skin and poor nail condition, and he certainly felt that he was in the second stage of the CFS disease process.

Very recent research has found strong evidence of elevated brain temperature in CFS patients[15]. This confirms the concept of brain inflammation, as described by the very old term myalgic encephalomyelitis.

Stage 3

Chronic fatigue becomes chronic fatigue syndrome

The second stage of the disease process can soon progress to the third stage, as a consequence of any viral infection. Examples of such infections include the common cold, influenza and glandular fever.

Therefore at this point, we have a state of chronic EFA deficiencies, occurring simultaneously with the presence of a hidden bacterial/microbial infection. If a viral infection is contracted at this time, conditions for the third stage of the CFS disease process will then be met.

This viral infection will now appear to become difficult to overcome and could last for some weeks. This occurs because the immune system is already dealing with the problems caused by possible EFA deficiencies, and a hidden infection (usually bacterial).

If left untreated, this condition will become chronic. This may occur gradually, over some months, or acutely over a few weeks. If it happens acutely, it will appear that it was triggered or started by influenza or some other common viral illness. This would explain why some cases of CFS happen when the patient contracts the flu and never seems to fully recover from its effects.

Frank's experience:

When Frank was diagnosed with CFS, he had been struggling with what was thought to be glandular fever. Tests for the Epstein Barr virus (EBV) came back negative, but the doctor's opinion was that he still had some sort of viral infection.

Frank had swollen lymph nodes – or glands – at the back of the neck, and he remembers that this was really unusual for him. In fact, he still can't recall another time when this had happened.

A strange feeling of exhaustion, or the special type of fatigue that is experienced in CFS, soon became evident.

Stage 4

Full CFS symptoms, with reactivation of dormant viruses

When this stage is reached, the patient will normally be at the point of being diagnosed with chronic fatigue syndrome. Given the fact that the preceding conditions have now been met, full CFS symptoms will now be in evidence.

Symptoms will vary in accordance to a number of factors including the levels of EFAs that are present in the body, together with the severity of the microbial/bacterial infection present. The triggering viral infection mentioned in the previous section will now have been substantially overcome.

Therefore, although patient will have overcome this viral infection, it will be soon obvious that all is not well. For the purpose of illustrating an example, we will refer to this infection as being a typical case of influenza.

Different symptoms will now start to emerge. It will appear that the bout of influenza that may have initially been experienced has returned. But instead of just being another case of influenza, a vague assortment of symptoms of other diseases may appear.

It is known that certain viruses such as those that cause childhood illnesses like chicken pox, measles, mumps and rubella are capable of persisting and remaining permanently within the body. It is only through the action of a healthy immune system that these do not normally reactivate. For example, the human herpes virus (HHV) that causes chicken pox may cause shingles, many years after the bout of chicken pox was initially overcome.

Patients may now experience partial reactivation of any number of viruses that have remained in the body. According to conventional medical thinking, such reactivation of viruses is very unusual. However, it is felt that in CFS this situation is normal as the immune system is already activated and malfunctioning.

It is believed that when researchers test chronic fatigue syndrome patients, and find a virus as a potential cause of CFS, it could be a reactivated virus that they have actually detected. This would explain why numerous viruses have been discovered, and yet no single infective agent has been determined to cause CFS.

Therefore, it seems that many researchers have been led astray in assuming that chronic fatigue syndrome must be caused by a specific virus. As viral reactivation can occur very intermittently during the course of a typical case of CFS, it is likely that no evidence of an active virus will be detected.

Indeed, medical attempts at detecting a source of infection

will usually be fruitless, with results of tests being almost completely normal.

This is because ordinary blood tests have not been sophisticated enough to detect what is causing the symptoms of chronic fatigue syndrome. However, the situation is changing with rapidly evolving medical technological advances.

As a consequence of not being able to detect the cause of CFS, some doctors have mistakenly formed the conclusion that this must therefore be is a psychological or psychiatric disorder. The authors of this book feel that this myth can finally be proved to be wrong.

Frank's experience:

When Frank had severe CFS symptoms, it is thought that he experienced the reactivation of two dormant viruses. In hindsight, it is now clear that the viruses that cause mumps and shingles were partially reactivated on an intermittent basis.

It is now evident that his immune system was acting-up and in obvious disarray. He had no reason to doubt that it was indeed malfunctioning, activated, and generally doing strange things.

Dental health and the immune response

It is difficult to believe how many CFS sufferers have had trouble with dental infections. The authors estimate that at least 90% have unusual types of gum diseases that refuse to heal properly. There is often some evidence of an infection, but this is usually ignored by dentists/doctors as there is little, if any, immune system response. This means that there is often no evidence of inflammation or discomfort.

Frank's experience:

While he was sick and not taking EFAs, Frank noticed that a cut finger would not get inflamed and took a very long time to heal. Dental problems such as a deep abscess also triggered no obvious immune system response.

The abscess was eventually overcome, after much trouble and many courses of antibiotics.

He had just received a thorough check-up and was finally been given the all clear by his dentist when Frank started taking large doses of EFAs. To his astonishment, he went on to have a newly apparent major gum infection. He had a near normal immune response together with obvious inflammation, a few weeks after he last saw the dentist!

The only plausible explanation for this was that the EFAs had somehow repaired Frank's immune system. This possibly explains why diseases, such as those due to staphylococci and mycoplasma infections, can remain totally hidden because of immune system problems.

Therefore, it is now apparent that the full extent of any infection usually remains hidden until proper EFA levels are able to repair the immune system response.

4

The situation changes

Since being diagnosed with CFS in 1994, Frank has experienced periods of incomplete remissions alternating with relapses. As mentioned earlier in this book, these apparent periods of recovery were not durable in their nature.

In other words, although they were times when he was relatively well CFS always seemed to be in the background.

Since 1998, Frank found that essential fatty acids were important to his health[1]. Later he found that resveratrol[14] was also helpful.

Unfortunately, fatigue continued to be a major problem. The best that could the achieved until September 2019 was about 9 hours of sleep and bedrest in a 24-hour period.

In recent years, Frank's health had deteriorated slowly and he was consistently needing 13 hours of sleep and bedrest in any 24-hour period.

In September 2019, Frank suffered a minor stroke and the situation changed dramatically. While recovering in hospital he was given stroke medication consisting of Atorvastatin SZ, Ado-perindopril and aspirin.

Somehow, the profound fatigue that he was experiencing began to disappear. Near the end of September, it had reduced to a point where only eight hours of sleep were required in any 24-hour period. No bedrest, apart from normal sleep, was now necessary.

This stunning situation resulted in Frank writing about his experience while searching for answers; how could some commonly available stroke medications have any influence on CFS?

The treatment of long term CFS using a high dose statin

The following is a summary of what Frank has learnt about his health since September 2019. It is hoped that this information might help others to improve their condition, although there are no guarantees. Everyone has a unique biochemistry and what might work for him might not work for anyone else.

Since starting treatment for an unrelated condition (the minor stroke), Frank has continued to recover from the devastating effects of CFS. The recovery process hasn't been instant and one wouldn't expect it to be.

It is only now that Frank truly realises how sick he really was, having struggled with crushing fatigue and immune disfunction since Christmas 1993.

Background information

Low cholesterol common in CFS

Dramatically low levels of pregnenolone is often found in long term CFS cases. Made from cholesterol, pregnenolone is the critical building block for steroid hormones such as estrogen and testosterone[8].

Interferon

In CFS, viral infections cause the body to make interferon in order to fight the infectious agent. This suppresses the mevalonic acid pathway that produces cholesterol and pregnenolone[8].

This is another reason for why widespread hormonal disorders are seen in CFS (along with the hypothalamic and gland dysfunction, and receptor resistance).

Low cholesterol or pregnenolone caused by infection

Acute infections respond well to interferon. However, this can lead to problems. Cholesterol blockers such as statins mildly block the same pathway and can actually have a mild antiviral effect at low dose (and a strong effect at high dose). These medications are used long term to treat high cholesterol. But they may starve the body of CoQ10 and pregnenolone and can, therefore cause CFS to flare up[8]. So it is suggested that statins should be taken with caution unless the body is given CoQ10 and pregnenolone supplements.

Frank is currently taking the following daily:

- 80mg Lipitor (atorvastatin).
- 50 to 100mg pregnenolone.
- 150 to 300 mg coenzyme Q10.
- 4 to 10 capsules of flax and/or fish oil because some people like Frank have greater than normal need for essential fatty acids. Evening primrose oil may occasionally be added.

The situation changes

It is very lucky that he was given the statin, atorvastatin as a routine post-stroke medication. In normal circumstances, Frank would not have had the chance to take this drug as it is a cholesterol lowering medication and he doesn't have high cholesterol. In fact, his level is on the low side of normal.

Statins exhibit broad antiviral properties on a dose dependent basis. Recently, it has been discovered that atorvastatin also acts as a probiotic and has other beneficial properties.

There is very little information about the treatment approach that Frank is using. Dr Jacob Teitelbaum has written about it and Frank considers him to be the world's leading expert on this topic[8].

For the latest studies about the many qualities of statins, or more specifically atorvastatin, it is suggested that the PubMed website (www.pubmed.gov) should be used. Our experience has demonstrated that it is a high-quality source of very detailed biomedical information.

Did olive leaf extract and other herbal supplements help the immune system to fully respond to atorvastatin?

Frank is still trying to fully understand his recovery from over two and a half decades of dealing with CFS.

Apart from the thoughts of Dr Teitelbaum, he has found very little to explain his dramatic return to good health.

One would have expected that other people would have found that atorvastatin was helpful in treating their CFS. Frank has been active in a very large online support forum, and his post detailing his remission has been viewed a vast number of times. However, he has been unable to find any examples of anyone admitting that statins have helped ease their chronic fatigue symptoms.

Moreover, an extensive search of the internet has failed to find anyone who has had a recovery similar to his. Perhaps, Frank's remission isn't solely due to this statin?

Herbal supplements

Maybe the olive leaf extract and other herbal supplements that Frank was taking immediately before his stroke prepared his immune system to work with atorvastatin to overcome CFS? The Memorial Sloan Kettering Cancer Center in the USA has excellent online information about these herbs and supplements[13].

Could it be that it was the combination of the things that Frank was taking that was the key factor in his recovery? Obviously, Frank had to stop taking them when he was in hospital.

Prior to being admitted to hospital, he was taking the following per day:

- Olive leaf extract (high strength) in powder form.

The situation changes

- Astragalus capsules (typical dosage).
- Echinacea capsules (2×5 gram capsules).
- Resveratrol caplets (high strength).
- Propolis capsules (high strength).
- Essential fatty acids (fish, flax and evening primrose oil).
- Garlic oil (1 to 4 capsules).

From what Frank has read, it can take about two weeks for vitamins and other supplements to be completely eliminated from the body[12].

So, one wonders if taking the above supplements together with atorvastatin would be a universally effective treatment regimen for CFS?

Unfortunately, there are no clinical trials (to the best of the authors' knowledge at time of writing) being carried out that might answer this question.

Frank Bartosy

5

My experience living with a CFS sufferer

The following is Nick's account of what it was like to grow up with a father who has a poorly understood and invisible chronic illness called CFS

It's difficult for me to talk about my dad's experience with CFS because I've barely known him without it. I was six years old when Dad got the flu. I only knew that it required lots of bedrest and that he should be better in a week or two. It didn't worry me, I was more concerned with what would happen at school the next day or choosing which Lego set to buy next.

Gradually it became obvious that Dad had passed the point where he should have been back to normal. Instead of recovering, the need for rest and quiet increased. Dad had been lucky enough to work from home, but this was no longer feasible. Family outings were nearly impossible even for a short time and distance. Other family members could and did fill in the gap, but Dad was stuck at home.

If you were lucky, he'd be able to have a brief chat after getting home as long as you kept the curtains closed and lights off.

Skip to September 2019. Dad has now been living with CFS to many varying degrees for 26 years. I found myself very late on a Saturday night in a hospital, looking at Dad who just had a stroke. The mind races to process this but doesn't seem to get very far. It seems so unfair. You know that there's always somebody worse off than you, but it doesn't make it any easier to handle when it happens to someone you know. You can offer physical and emotional support but ultimately, you feel very powerless.

Recovering from a stroke would be bad enough, but CFS complicates it so much. The routine that Dad could control at home is now thrown into a state of constant high alert. In the hospital, there are no windows to enable you to tell day from night. Nurses and patients can make noise at any time. CFS isn't well understood at the best of times but in this environment it just can't be accommodated for, even with the best of intentions.

Despite all of this, over the next few days Dad seemed to be doing really well. You try not to get your hopes up too much, but this is what keeps you going. Amazingly about a week later, Dad seemed well enough to go home. He and I both knew that the lack of quality rest since the start of his hospital stay was affecting him. It was hard to know whether many of his symptoms were caused by CFS or the stroke, but leaving hospital seemed to be the only way to find out for sure.

It was a relief when Dad got home and could control his routine again. Progress is of course slow at first, and in the back of your mind you wonder if things will stay this way forever or get worse. After a few days, it seemed that Dad couldn't sleep anywhere near his normal amount at home. It looked like insomnia, except that his need to rest during the day seemed to be gone as well. He gradually took back control of his routine.

Half a year later, Australia braces itself for a global pandemic and rapidly comes to terms with the need to isolate. It feels like Dad has been preparing for this for nearly half his life and has finally made it through to the other side.

Conclusion

At the time of writing, it is evident that only a very small percentage of CFS sufferers have achieved what could be considered to be a durable remission.

It is our sincere wish that all CFS patients are able to find what works for them and consequently regain a state of robust health.

We also hope that a universally accepted diagnostic test for CFS can finally be developed. The previously stated concept of diagnosis based on symptoms alone is liable to result in cases of misdiagnosis. The other problem is that if someone's condition improves, there is no definite way to tell whether or not he/she still has the illness to some degree.

Finally, Frank would like to mention that he is feeling like he used to before contracting CFS in 1994. He is getting his life back together and it is uncanny how good being healthy again actually feels. In addition, Frank is still working on improving his physical fitness and practicing taekwondo patterns on most days.

One consequence of having CFS for a very long time is that he has become much more of a spiritual person than before his illness began. He is profoundly grateful to God for helping him to achieve a durable remission from CFS.

References

1. Bartosy F. Victory over *Chronic Fatigue Syndrome*. Australia: Seaview Press; 1998.

2. Bartosy F. *Newcastle tests explained* (website). Melbourne, Australia: CFS and FMS Research; 1999. For more info about the edited and simplified articles, please contact the authors of this book via the publisher.

3. Shepherd C. *Living with ME*. Great Britain: Cedar. 1992.

4. McGregor N., *An Omic Analysis of ME/CFS: An assessment of potential mechanisms.* https://mecfsconference.org.au/videos/neil-mcgregor/

5. Newberry F., Hsieh S.Y., Wileman T., Carding S.R.,: *Does the microbiome and virome contribute to myalgic encephalomyelitis/chronic fatigue syndrome?* Clin Sci (Lond) 15 March 2018; 132 (5): 523–542. doi: https://doi.org/10.1042/CS20171330

6. Vocapture. Offline Englishdictionary app. for Android. Ontario, Canada 2020.

7. Nagy-Szakal D., Williams, B.L., Mishra, N., et al. *Fecal metagenomic profiles in subgroups of patients with myalgic encephalomyelitis/chronic fatigue syndrome.* Microbiome 5, 44 (2017). https://doi.org/10.1186/s40168-017-0261-y

8. Teitelbaum, J. MD. *Exciting New Discovery in Treating CFS & Fibromyalgia.* New York, NY May 2011. https://www.psychologytoday.com/au/blog/complementary-medicine/201105/exciting-new-discovery-in-treating-cfs-fibromyalgia

9. CDC (Centers for Disease Control and Prevention). *Chronic fatigue syndrome: 1994 case definition.* 2012. [December 16, 2013]. http://www.cdc.gov/cfs/case-definition/1994.html . [Reference list]

10. Committee on the Diagnostic Criteria for Myalgic Encephalomyelitis/Chronic Fatigue Syndrome; Board on the Health of Select Populations; Institute of Medicine. Beyond Myalgic Encephalomyelitis/Chronic Fatigue Syndrome: Redefining an Illness. Washington (DC): National Academies Press (US); 2015 Feb 10. 3, Current Case Definitions and Diagnostic Criteria, Terminology, and Symptom Constructs and Clusters. Available from: https://www.ncbi.nlm.nih.gov/books/NBK284898/

11. Eramus U. *Fats that heal and fats that kill* Canada: Alive Books.

References

12. Rahm, D. MD, *A Guide to Perioperative Nutrition*, Aesthetic Surgery Journal, Volume 24, Issue 4, July 2004, Pages 385–390, https://doi.org/10.1016/j.asj.2004.04.001

13. Memorial Sloan Kettering Cancer Center, New York, NY 10065 (website). See https://www.mskcc.org/cancer-care/diagnosis-treatment/symptom-management/integrative-medicine/herbs/search

14. *Resveratrol could counter metabolic diseases,* animal study (article on the internet). By staff reporter. 2006. See https://www.nutraingredients.com/Article/2006/12/15/Resveratrol-could-counter-metabolic-diseases-animal-study

15. Younger, J. PhD, *How Brain Inflammation Causes ME/CFS.* (video on the internet). 2018. https://youtu.be/8XrdSlpUQTE

Index

A

aches, 10-11

antibiotics, 36

astragalus, 45

atorvastatin, 40, 42-44, 46

B

bacterial, 24, 29-30, 31-33

bedrest, 17-19, 39-40, 47

Bioscreen, 3, 8-9, 25

blood tests, 30, 35

brain fog, 19, 25

brain inflammation, 31, 55

    temperature, 31

C

cfids, 7, 11

cholesterol, 41-43

circadian rhythm(s), 18

circulation, 28

conventional medical thinking, 34

cytokines, 29-30

D

dental

    abscess, 31

    health, 36

E

echinacea, 45

energy, 17-20

Epstein-Barr virus, 10, 14

evening primrose oil, 43, 45

exhaustion, 10-11, 17-18, 33

F

fever, 10, 31

    glandular, 9-10, 31-32

fish oil, 1, 43, 45

flax oil, 1, 43, 45

G

garlic, 45

gastrointestinal flora, 22, 25

    symptoms, 11

genome(s), 22-23

glandular fever, 9-10, 31-32

glucose tolerance, 24

gut barrier, 23

    bacteria, 26

I
immune system(s), 11, 23, 27, 29-30, 32, 34-37, 44

infection(s), 8, 10, 12, 15, 26-33, 35-37, 41-42

inflammation, 27-28, 31, 36-37, 55

    brain, 31, 55

influenza, 9, 19, 31-34

interferon, 41-42

L
lie down, 18

lipid metabolism, 24

Lipitor, 42

liver, 30

lymphokines, 29-30

lymph nodes, 10, 32

M

microbial infection(s), 10, 29, 32-33

microbiome, 23-24, 53-54

myalgia, 8

myalgic encephalomyelitis, 7, 15, 31, 53-54

myelin, 24

N

nutritional deficiencies, 27

O

oil

    evening primrose, 1, 43, 45

    fish, 1, 43, 45

    flax, 1, 43, 45

olive leaf, 44-45

P

pregnenolone, 41-42

probiotics, 22, 25

propolis, 45

psychiatric disorder, 35

R

reactivation of viruses, 33-35

rest, 17, 47-49

resveratrol, 39, 45, 55

S

skin, 11, 28, 31

sleep, 18, 39-40, 49

staphylococci, 30, 37

supplements, 42, 44-46

T

taekwondo, 1, 52

temperature, 30-31

toxin(s), 23, 30

V

viral reactivation, 34

    infection(s), 26, 31-33, 41

virome, 23-24, 53

vitamin F, 27

W

walking, 18

www.ingramcontent.com/pod-product-compliance
Lightning Source LLC
Chambersburg PA
CBHW071727020426
42333CB00017B/2420